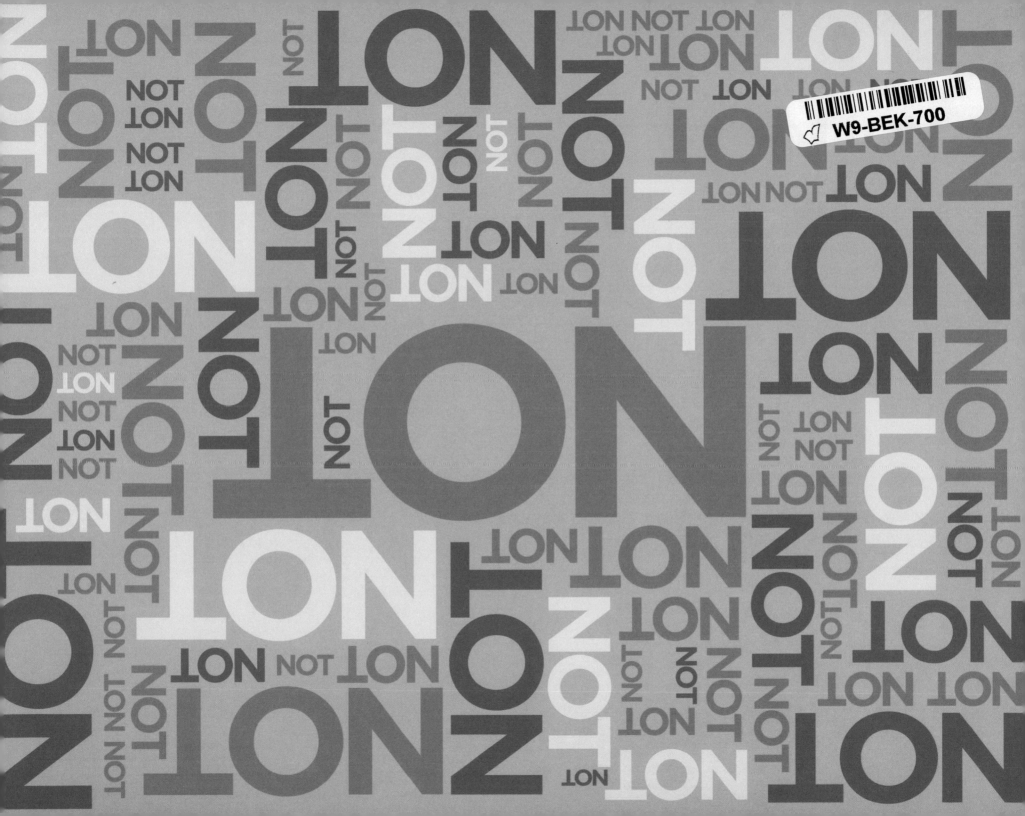

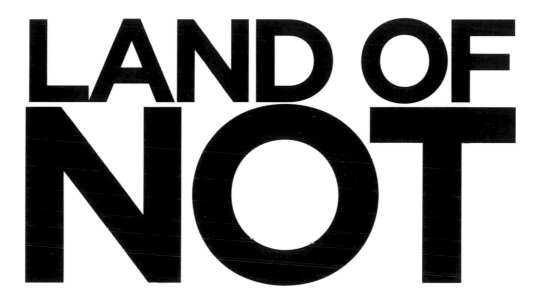

LAND OF NOT

NOT THE ILLUSTRATOR : J.J. VULOPAS

NOT THE AUTHOR : BILL DUSSINGER

Lancaster, Pa

Written by J.J. Vulopas
Illustrations by Bill Dussinger

Printed in the United States of America

ISBN: 978-0-9993845-0-3 (Hardcover)
        978-0-9993845-1-0 (Paperback)

For information:
717-205-3856
www.thelandofcan.com, www.citizensofcan.com
jj@thelandofcan.com

Citizens Of Can
1060 Manheim Pike
Lancaster PA 17601

LAND OF NOT

NOT THE ILLUSTRATOR : J.J. VULOPAS

NOT THE AUTHOR : BILL DUSSINGER

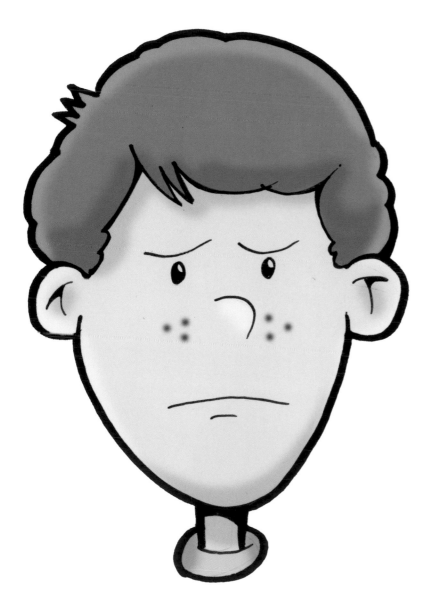

Once upon a time in the **Land of Not**, there was a boy who could **not** eat nuts.

His name was **not** Johnny or Randy or Paul. He was **not** 47 or 5 or 95. And he was **not** happy because he could **not** eat nuts.

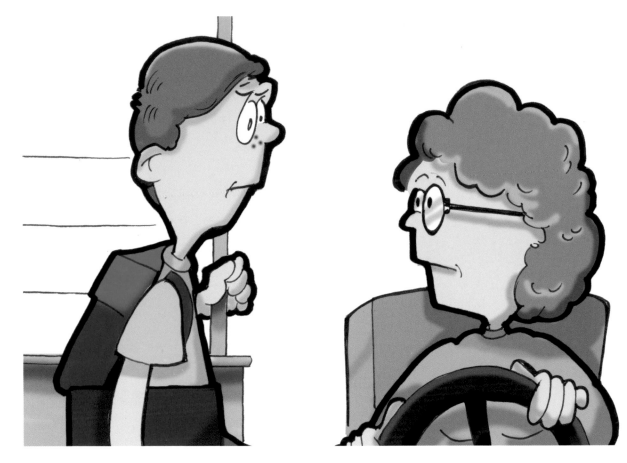

"Hi, kid who **can't** eat nuts," said a woman who was **not** driving a green boat or a　　　truck or a pink train. "You do **not** look happy today."

"Hi, **not** Mrs. Smith," said the boy as he sat in his assigned seat, which was **not** in the front or at a window. "You do **not** look happy either."

Indeed, both were **frowning**.

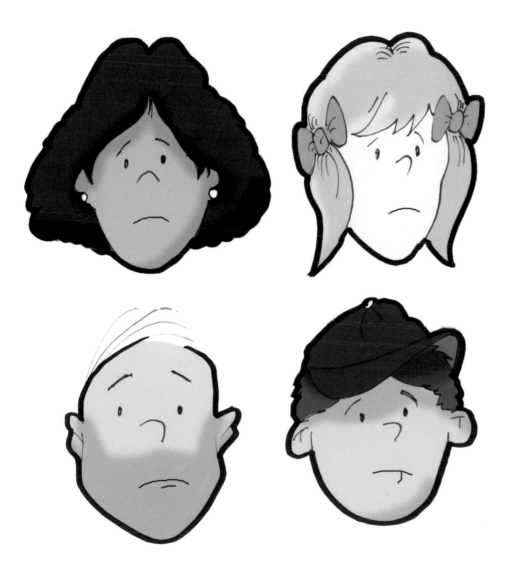

You see, in the **Land of Not** people were known by what they were **not**. By what they **couldn't** do, by what they **didn't** do, by what they **didn't** like.

And everyone was **not** happy.

"I **don't** like the violin."

"I **don't** speak Spanish."

"I **can't** see clearly without my glasses."

"I'm **not** Jackie."

Every day that was **not** Saturday or Sunday, the woman who was **not** Mrs. Smith took the students to a building that was **not** a post office or a restaurant or a movie theater. And every day, the students repeated the same chant along the way:

"I am a kid from the **Land of Not**! I **cannot**, know **not**, do **not**, am **not**!"

"I am a kid from the **Land of Not**! I **cannot**, know **not**, do **not**, am **not**!"

"I am a kid from the **Land of Not**! I **cannot**, know **not**, do **not**, am **not**!"

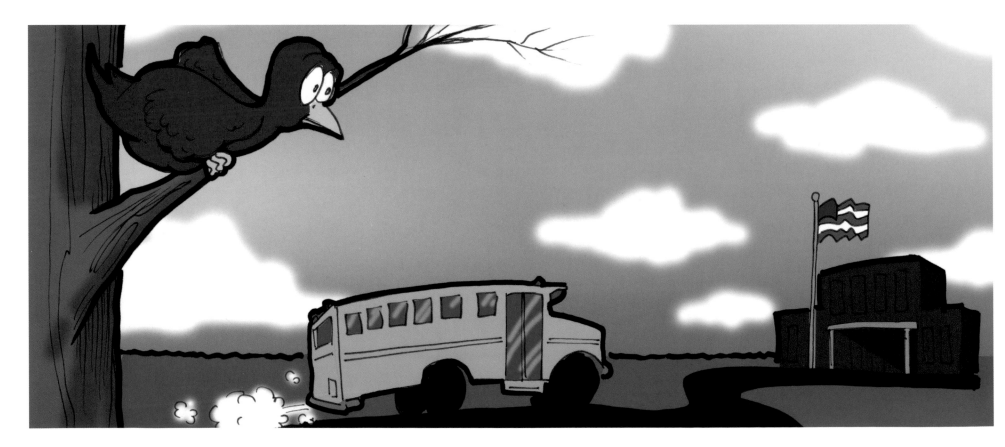

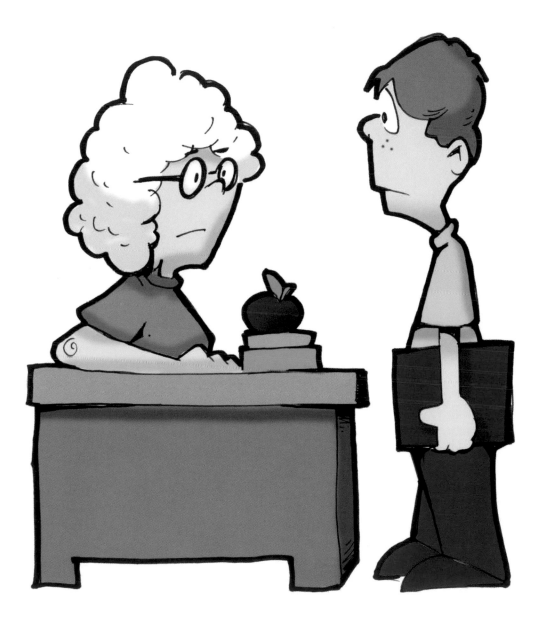

It was another dreary day in the **Land of Not**. Every day was **not** sunny. The bus arrived at the building.

"Hello, boy who **can't** eat nuts," sulked the woman who did **not** teach reading or science or history.

As the students took their seats in the classroom, a man who was **not** wearing sneakers or shorts walked in with a new student.

NOT PAGE 582

"Hello, class," said the man. "This boy's name is **not** Henry or Roy and he's **not** from the **Land of Not**. He does **not** live on Walnut Street, he does **not** have a dog, his favorite color is **not** green, and he does **not** know how to draw."

"I **can't** draw either," moped the girl in the front row.

"Perfect. You two will make great friends," he said while giving her a **thumbs down**. "Let's all introduce ourselves. Boy who **can't** throw a football, you go first."

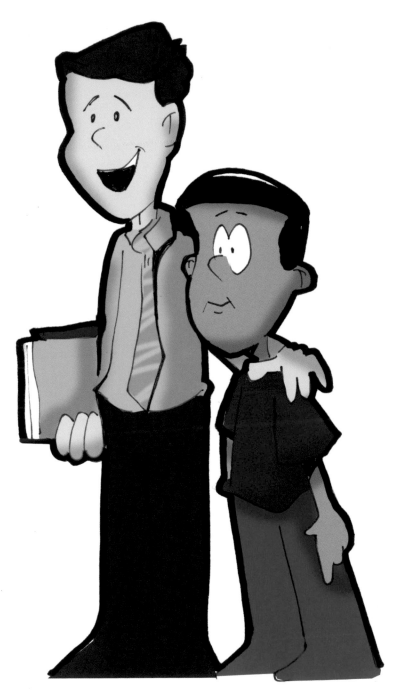

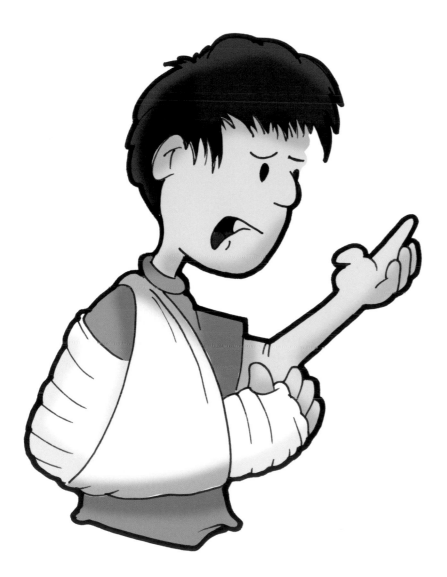

The boy in the front whose arm was in a sling stood up.

"My name is **not** Simon or Sally or Sam," he said with a **frown**. "I **can't** play sports right now. I **don't** know how to cook eggs, and I **don't** like yellow."

NOT PAGE TRIANGLE

The girl in the second row stood next.

"Hi, boy who **doesn't** like green. My name is **not** Anna, I **can't** read Russian, and my birthday is **not** March 12 or March 19 or October 4."

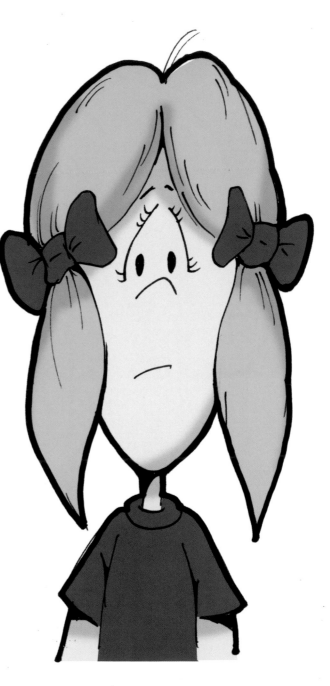

NOT PAGE 71

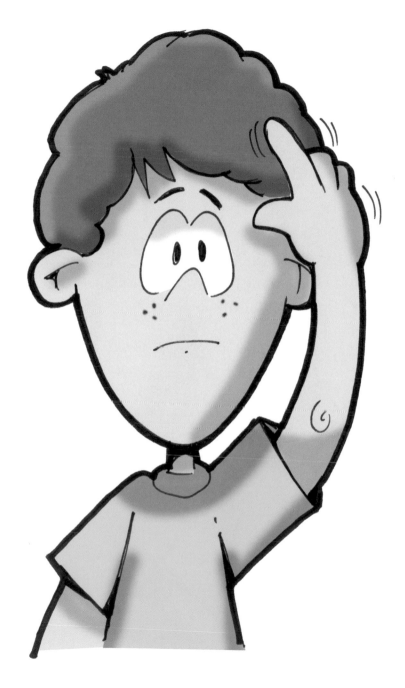

"My birthday is **not** October 4, either," said the boy in the back, whom we met at the start of this story. He stood and spoke.

"My name is **not** Gary or Michael. I've never visited Tokyo, I **can't** eat nuts, and I **don't** know my times tables."

NOT PAGE 134

The teacher stood from her desk. "Boy who is **not** from **Not**, you can sit beside the girl who **can't** ride a skateboard."

Though he **didn't** say it, the boy who was **not** from **Not** was confused about the **Land of Not** because no one smiled. **Not** the students, or the teacher, or the principal. A few minutes later another boy in the class raised his hand and announced to the teacher, "I really, really, really, really **don't** have to go to the bathroom right now."

"Okay," the teacher said. "I **don't** either."

The boy sat back down and the teacher continued the lesson.

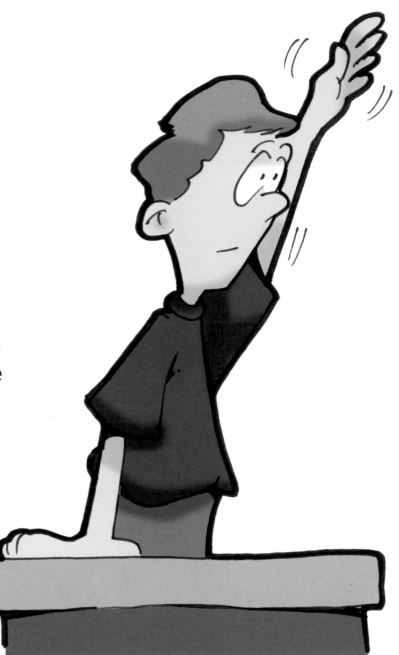

 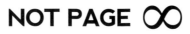

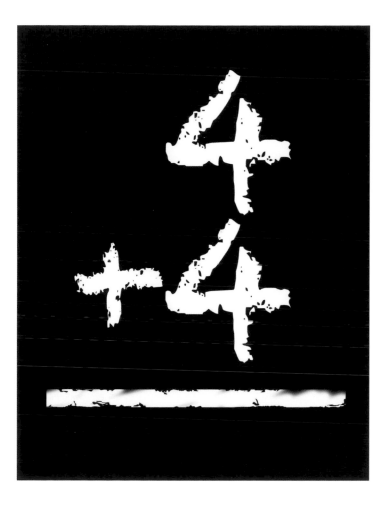

"What's 4 plus 4?" the teacher asked.

"**Not** 15!" shouted the girl in the front.

"Correct," the teacher said, writing NOT 15 on the board. "What else is it?"

"**Not** 127," shouted another student.

"Correct," said the teacher. "Boy **not** from **Not**, you haven't spoken yet. What's 4 plus 4?"

The boy who was **not** from **Not** looked around. Everyone was staring at him.

"Eight?" he said shyly.

"Eight?" the teacher repeated as the class chuckled. "Math is **not** a joke."

The boy could tell the teacher was **not** happy, and he **didn't** speak for the rest of the day.

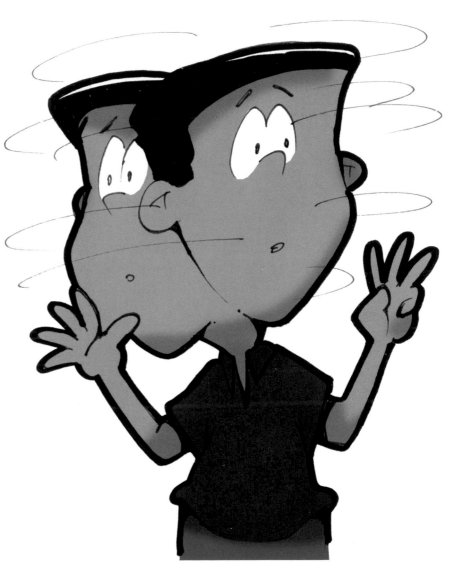

ERROR 404: PAGE NOT FOUND

The next day, which was **not** Wednesday, was show and tell day. The boy who was **not** named Bobby walked to the front of the room and held up a round ball.

"This is **not** a tennis racket," he said, as the class nodded. "I **can't** play tennis."

Next was a girl whose hair was **not** blonde.

"This is **not** a violin," she said holding up a metal instrument with a horn on the end of it. "I **can't** play string instruments."

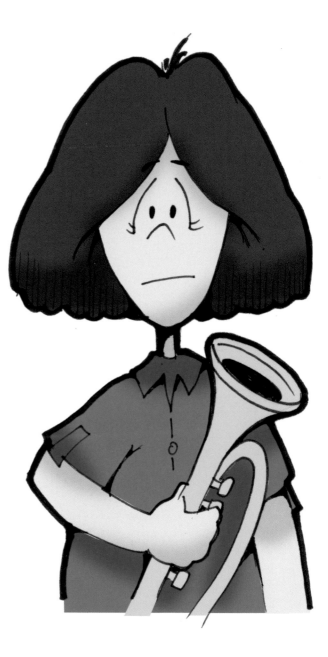

NOT PAGE 3.14159265358979323846264338327950288419716939937510582...

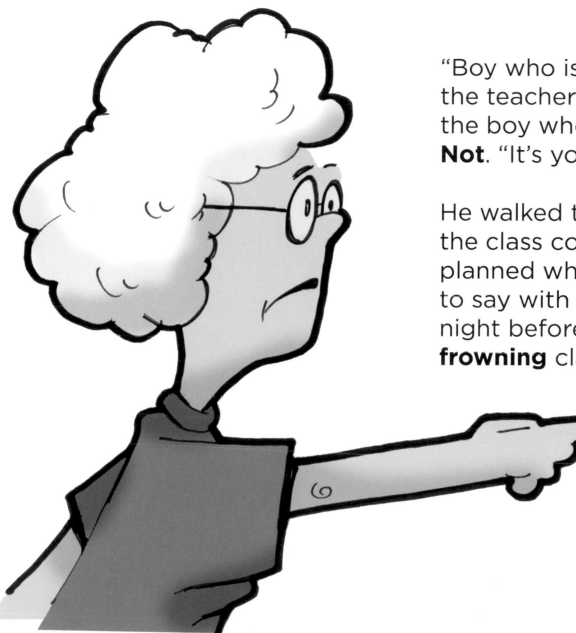

"Boy who is **not** Paul or Joe," the teacher said, pointing to the boy who was **not** from **Not**. "It's your turn."

He walked to the front of the class confidently. He had planned what he was going to say with his parents the night before. He looked at his **frowning** classmates.

... 0974944592307816406286208998628034825342117067982148086513282306

"Hi everyone. My name is **not** Paul or Joe," he said. "My name is **not** Jack or Jill or Rob or Red, and I could stand up here for the rest of the day telling you all of the names that are **not** mine. My name IS Collin."

The class gasped. The teacher jumped from her chair.

"Show and tell is **not** a joke," she said, her voice rising.

"Do you understand, boy who is **not** from the **Land of Not**?"

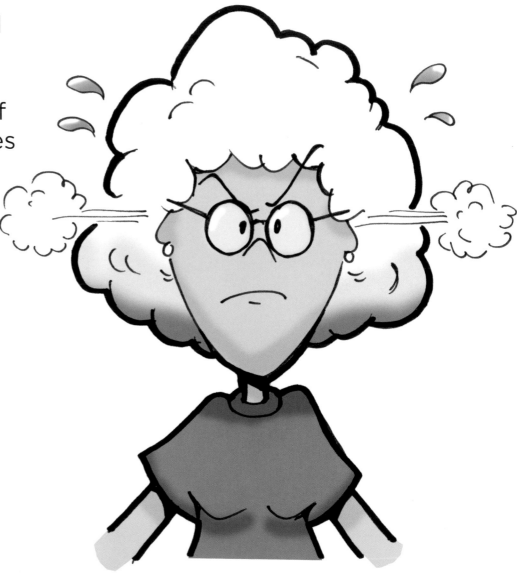

NOT PAGE 438

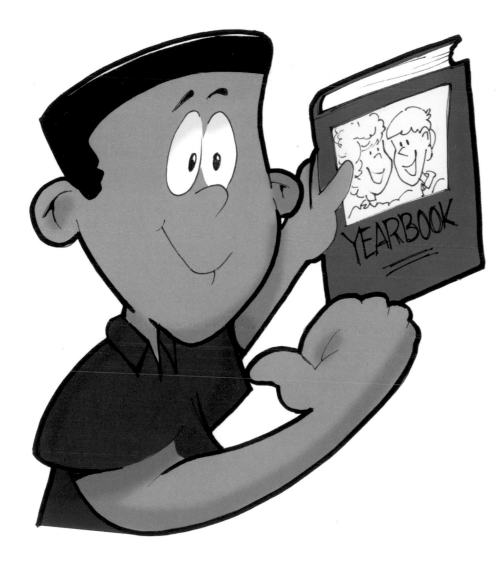

"My name **IS** Collin, and I'm from the **Land of Can**," he said. "In the **Land of Can**, I **can**. I **know**. I **do**. I **am**." He held up his old school's yearbook. "In these pages are my friends from the **Land of Can**."

The class was shocked because the kids on the cover of the yearbook were **not** frowning. They were **smiling**.

"Why are they **not** sad?" one student asked.

As Collin opened the book to the first page, the teacher ran from the room to get the principal.

"They are **happy**," Collin announced. "They are **happy** because they are doing what they **love**... they are being who they **are**." Collin pointed out different pictures in the yearbook. "Look," Collin said. "This boy is playing baseball because that's what he **likes**." He turned the page.

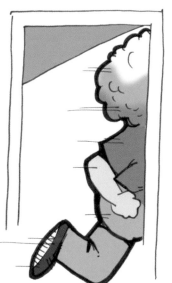

"And she is playing the violin. And she is coding a computer program."

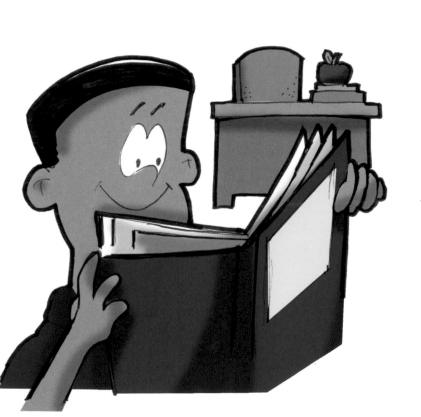

He closed the yearbook. "In the **Land of Can**, you don't know people based on what they're **not**."

NOT PAGE 12

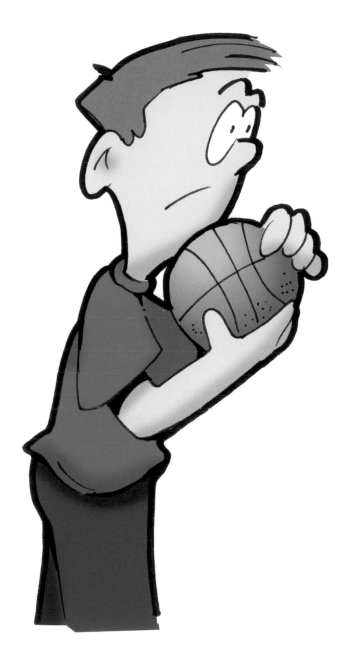

"You mean you **are** who you **are**?" one student asked.

"**Not** who you're **not**?" asked another.

"Exactly," Collin said, walking over to the boy holding a basketball.

"We **are** who we **are**, **not** who we're **not**."

Collin looked at the boy and smiled. "Who cares if you **can't** play tennis? This is **not** a tennis racket. It's a basketball, and you play basketball."

The boy stood still for a moment, then started dribbling the basketball slowly on the ground in front of him. *Bounce. Bounce bounce. Bounce bounce bounce.*

"You **can** do it!" Collin encouraged, and the class joined in. Soon, the boy was dribbling the ball like a pro, *bounce* between his legs, and *bounce bounce* over his head and *bounce bounce bounce bounce bounce* around his back, and the class **cheered**, and the boy **smiled**.

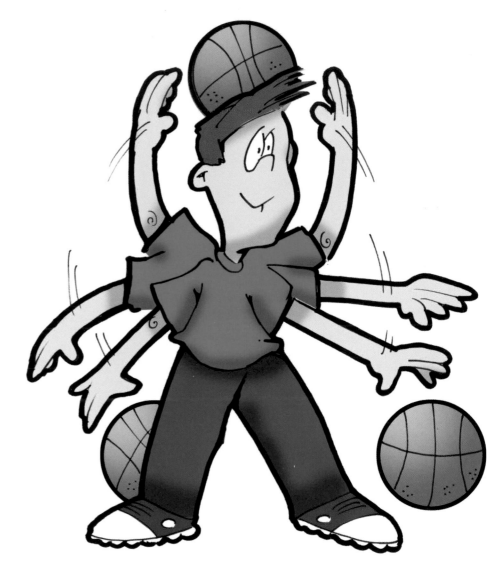

NOT PAGE 12

The cheers grew **louder** as the bounces bounced **higher** and **faster**. The class could be heard throughout the hallways.

Soon the teacher returned with the man who was **not** wearing sneakers. The students **stopped** cheering as the basketball dribbled to a stop. *Bounce bounce bounce. Bounce bounce. Bounce.*

"What's going on here?" the man who was **not** wearing sneakers demanded. "This is **not** how you should behave. This is **not** how it's supposed to be. This is **not** who we are in the **Land of Not**.

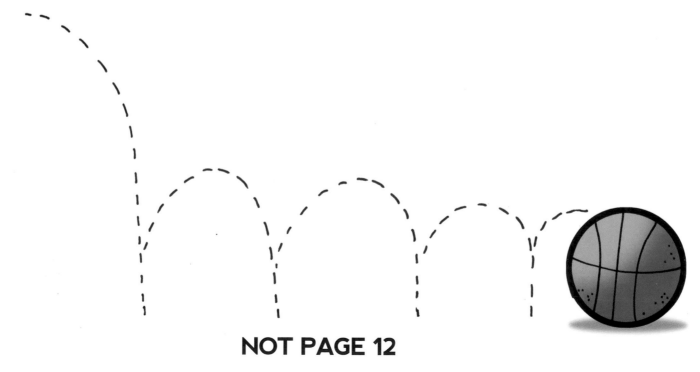

NOT PAGE 12

"Principal Handy," said a girl from the third row, calling him by his name. "My name is Claire and I **like** to play the trumpet." Claire held up her trumpet and played a beautiful tune.

Principal Handy could **not** believe what he was seeing.

The teacher just shook her head.

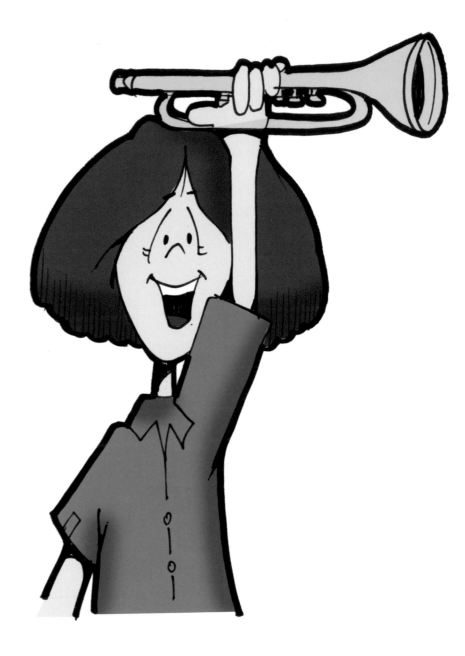

NOT PAGE PURPLE

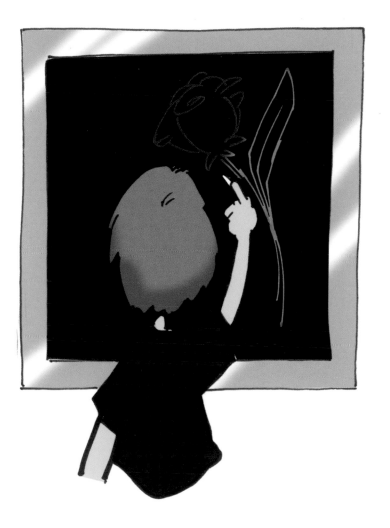

Then Bobby stood. "My name is Bobby and I **like** to draw!"

Bobby walked to the chalkboard. It was finally his chance to show his talent to someone other than his parents. He drew a red rose on the board and underneath it wrote the words "red rose."

NOT PAGE $\int \sqrt{x^3 + 1}\, dx$

The other students continued to **show their talents**. Morgan made a coin appear from behind Michael's ear, and Michael did a handstand in front of John's desk, and John started writing a rap about everything he was seeing, about all his friends, about all the talents, about all the **smiles**.

Everyone was **smiling**. Everyone, that is, **but** one.

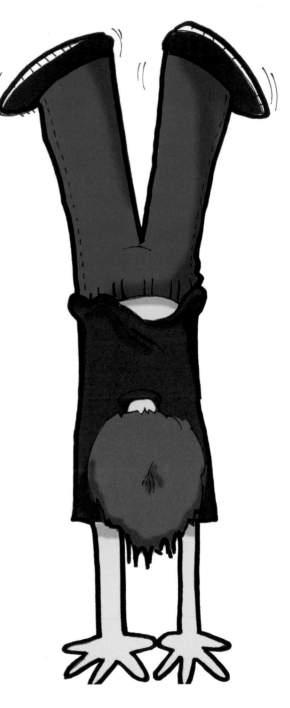

NOT PAGE GOOGOL

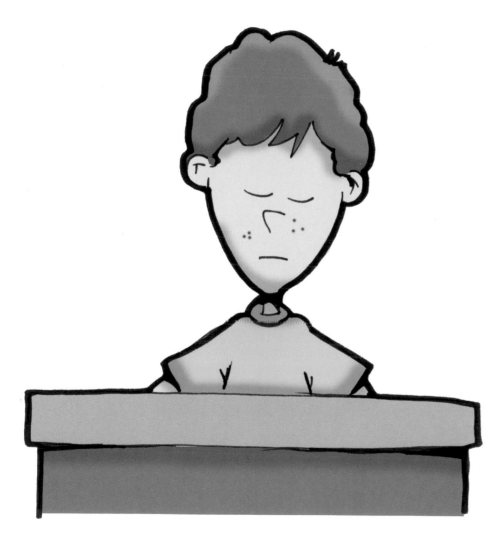

Collin looked to the back of the room and saw the boy who could **not** eat nuts sitting at his desk, **frowning**. Collin approached him. "What's wrong?" Collin asked. "Aren't you excited to show us who you are? You are more than the boy who **can't** eat nuts."

"This is all great," said the boy, "but people need to know that I **can't** eat nuts. If I eat nuts I could get really sick."

NOT PAGE 91

Collin put his hand on the boy's shoulder.

"Everybody has things that they **can't** do. I **can't** hear without my hearing aid. No one should ignore these things. We should **accept** them and **understand** them because they **are** very important. But we should **not** let them define us, and we certainly should **not** let them keep us sad."

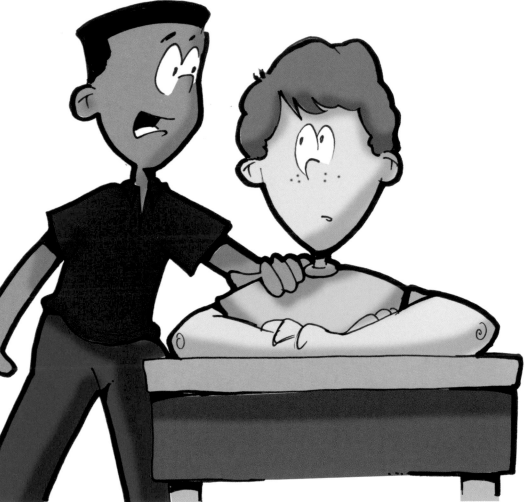

NOT PAGE 18

Behind them, the students were showing their skills and flipping through Collin's yearbook.

"I **can** take good pictures, too!" James said, pointing to a picture of a student with a camera.

"And I **like** helping animals!" Debbie said, turning to a picture of a field trip to the zoo.

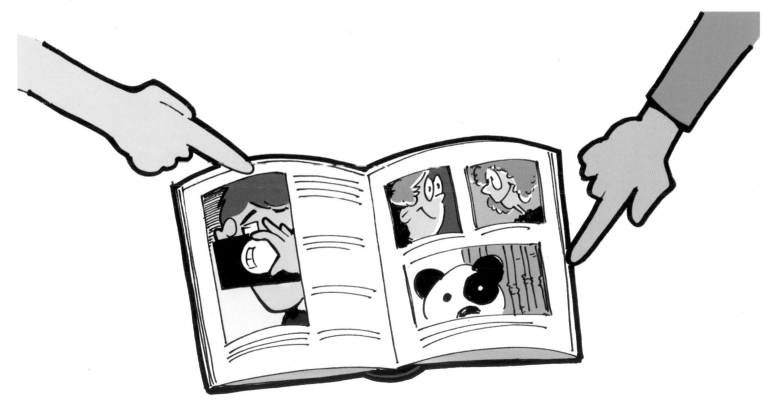

NOT PAGE 6.02 x 10^-23

Finally the boy who could **not** eat nuts stood on his desk. "Everybody!" he shouted. The students stopped talking and turned to face him. Even the principal and the teacher listened to what he had to say.

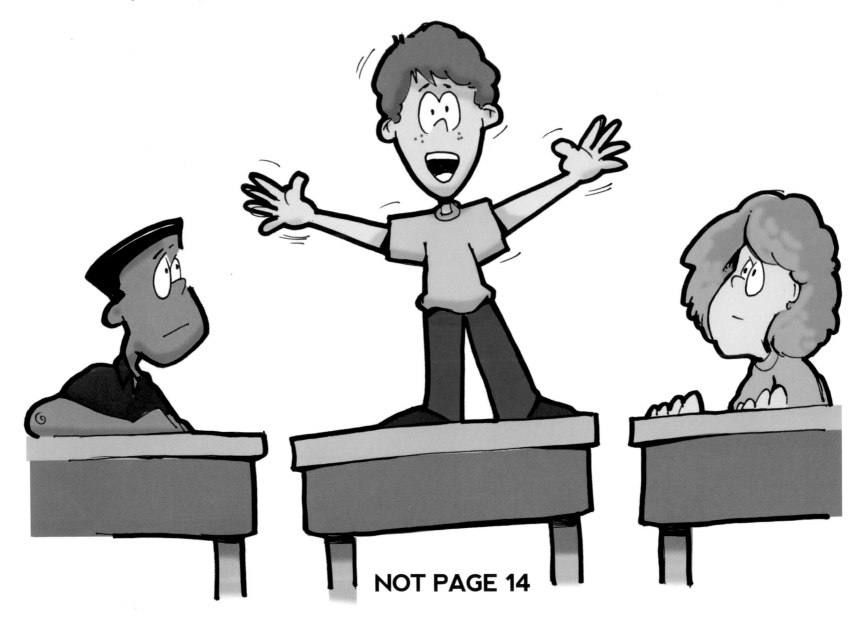

NOT PAGE 14

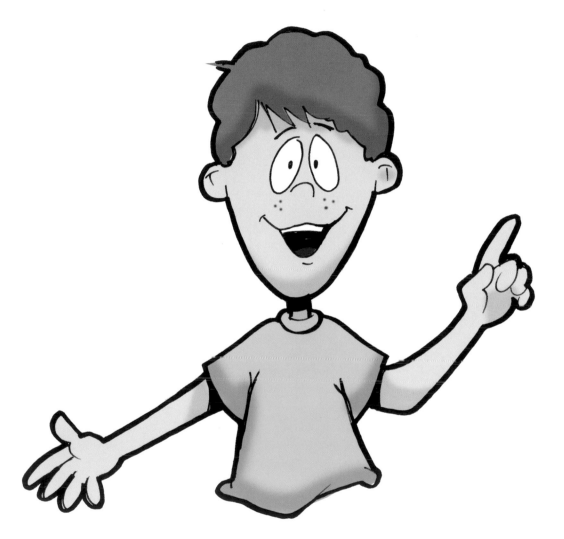

"My name is Tom. No, I **can't** eat nuts because they will get me really sick. It's important that you know that I **can't** eat nuts so you **can** be safe around me, but I don't want you to know me only as the boy who **can't** eat nuts. I want you to know me as the boy who **can** tell jokes and **can** run fast and **can** play chess."

A smile began to form on Tom's face. "I also want you to know me as the boy who **can** sing."

NOT PAGE 1

As the sun emerged from the clouds and **brightened** the classroom, Tom took a deep breath, looked at his **smiling** classmates, and **sang**:

"Do what you love.
Embrace what you've got.
You are who you are.
Not who you're not."

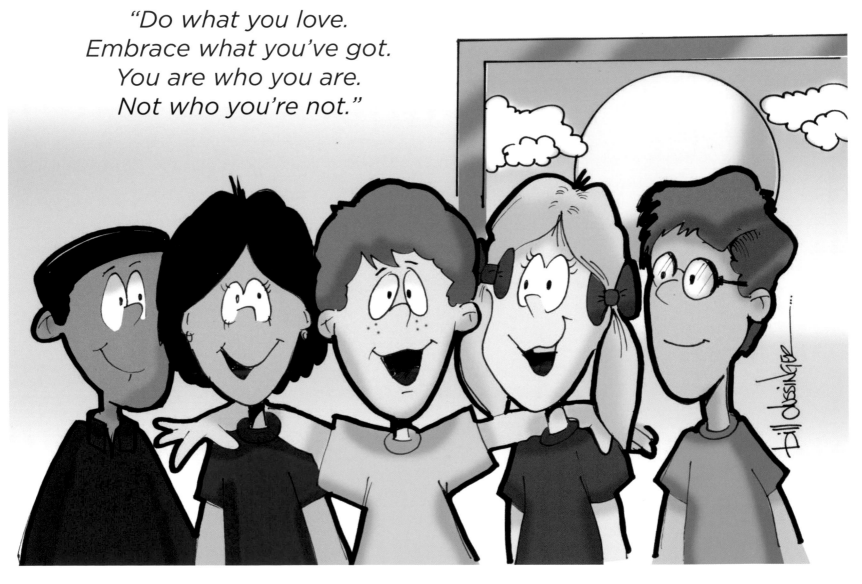

About the Author

JJ Vulopas can **not** drink milk or eat tree nuts... Oh, wait, we're living in the **Land of Can.** JJ is a 2019 graduate of the Wharton School of the University of Pennsylvania and lives in New York City. He is an advocate for young people, speaking across the nation about the top issues facing youth. He likes to play the piano, write computer programs, do math, travel, and read. He firmly believes that more is possible when young people define themselves by their strengths instead of their deficits.

Check out www.thelandofcan.com to see JJ's food allergy blog and www.citizensofcan.com to learn more about developing a CAN mindset. JJ can be contacted directly at jj@thelandofcan.com.

About the Illustrator

Bill Dussinger can **not** eat shellfish or take aspirin... He **can** draw fun illustrations for books like this one. He's been an illustrator, cartoonist and graphic designer for over 35 years. Bill has his own graphic design business, called Penny Lane Graphics (www.plgraphics.com). He is also a part time college instructor teaching graphic design and illustration at the Pennsylvania College of Art & Design. He can be contacted at bill@plgraphics.com.

Why red sneakers?

Hey, readers. It's JJ, the author of this book. Did you notice that many of the characters in *Land of Not* are wearing red sneakers? Did you wonder why?

Like Tom, one of the characters in the book, I have a food allergy. I can't drink milk or eat tree nuts. If I do, I can get very sick. It's serious. Because of my allergy, I work closely with some amazing food allergy organizations. One organization I love is Red Sneakers for Oakley, which raises awareness about the dangers of food allergies. The organization was founded in memory of Oakley Debbs who had a food allergy and who loved to wear his red sneakers wherever he went. His parents and sister started Red Sneakers for Oakley. They want everyone to know how serious food allergies are! To find out more about food allergies, please ask an adult or visit www.redsneakers.org

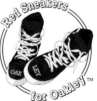

Do you know the 13 Words of Can?

Turn the page...

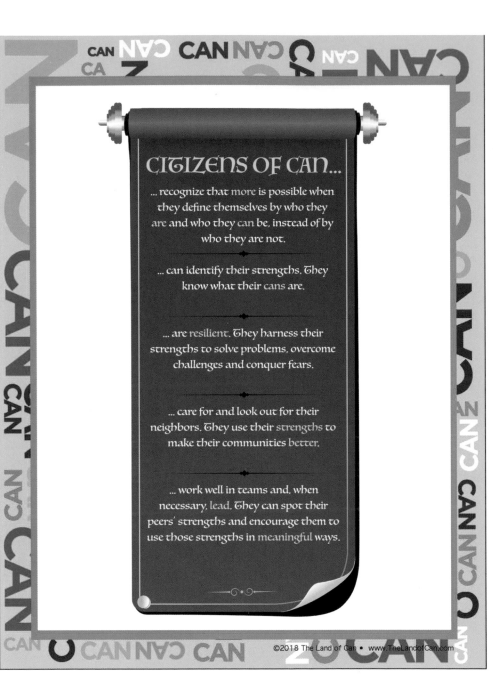

CAN Constitution

Collin and his friends from the Land of Can live by the principles outlined in the Can Constitution. By following these five tenets, you too can be a Citizen of Can.

Words of CAN

Collin & his friends know the 13 Words of CAN. How many of the CAN words do you know?

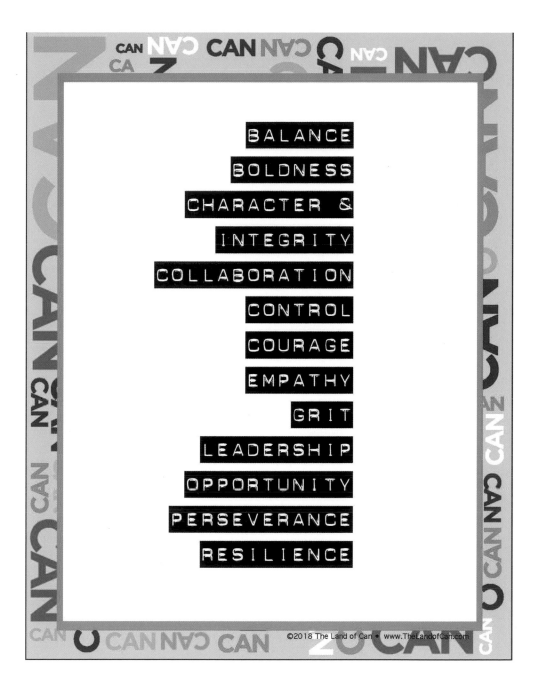

BALANCE
BOLDNESS
CHARACTER &
INTEGRITY
COLLABORATION
CONTROL
COURAGE
EMPATHY
GRIT
LEADERSHIP
OPPORTUNITY
PERSEVERANCE
RESILIENCE

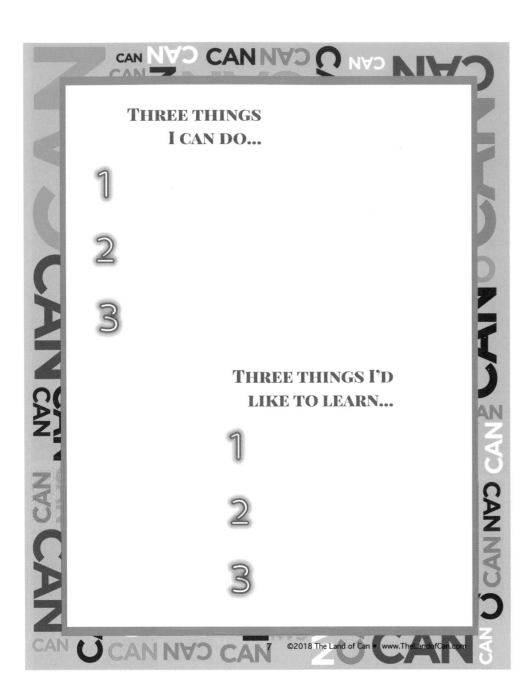

**THREE THINGS
I CAN DO...**

1

2

3

**THREE THINGS I'D
LIKE TO LEARN...**

1

2

3

What can you do? What would you like to learn how to do?

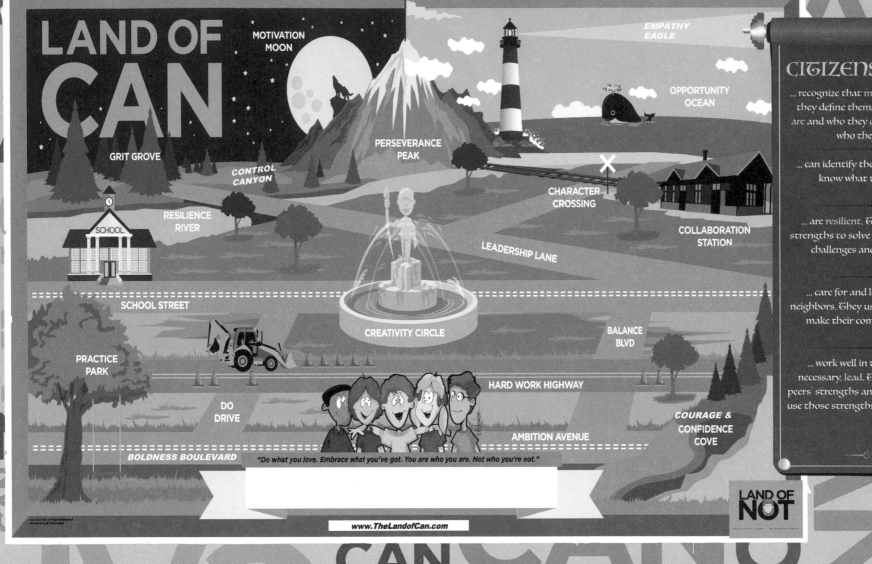

LAND OF CAN

MOTIVATION MOON

EMPATHY EAGLE

OPPORTUNITY OCEAN

PERSEVERANCE PEAK

GRIT GROVE

CONTROL CANYON

CHARACTER CROSSING

RESILIENCE RIVER

SCHOOL

COLLABORATION STATION

LEADERSHIP LANE

SCHOOL STREET

CREATIVITY CIRCLE

BALANCE BLVD

PRACTICE PARK

DO DRIVE

HARD WORK HIGHWAY

COURAGE & CONFIDENCE COVE

AMBITION AVENUE

BOLDNESS BOULEVARD

"Do what you love. Embrace what you've got. You are who you are. Not who you're not."

CITIZENS OF CAN...

... recognize that more is possible when they define themselves by who they are and who they can be, instead of by who they are not.

... can identify their strengths. They know what their cans are.

... are resilient. They harness their strengths to solve problems, overcome challenges and conquer fears.

... care for and look out for their neighbors. They use their strengths to make their communities better.

... work well in teams and, when necessary, lead. They can spot their peers' strengths and encourage them to use those strengths in meaningful ways.

LAND OF NOT